Practical guide for anesthesia

Author: Hala Mostafa Goma ,MD,professor of anesthesia ,Faculty of medicine,Cairo University

Ahmeda1995@yahoo.com

3834Table of contents:

Introduction   3

Skills and practice 4

Anesthetist health: 5

safety and quality   6

Basic Anesthesia Machine Set-Up Checklist   8
Safe anesthesia during radiologic investigations   9

Anesthesiologist patient relation ship   12
Anesthesia team work   14

career and financial aspects of anesthesiologist: 16

Preoperative preparation   17

Preoperative Anesthesia Machine Checklist Recommendations   25

Pacemaker and implantable cardioverter defibrillator   27

Monitoring   27

Intraoperative fluid management   30

Intra operative special anesthesia techniques   32

Ultrasonographic nerve blochade   34

Preparation and check list for peripheral nerve blockade   35

Skills needed for cardiothoracic   37

Postoperative management: 38

Suggested reading   40

Introduction:

Anesthesia is a very important specialty. Safety of patients is the main requirement, and it is the aim of every anesthesiologist. It is an art, includes safety measures for our patients, continuous learning, acquiring new skills, training of young anesthesiologists, and research work. Anesthesia is a Working within an anesthesia team, sharing work, and good partnership inside and outside the operating room. Encourage each other, continuous support, learning, and advices from the senior staff for the junior staff it will be as one family, this relation makes advantages for patients safety, decreasing stress, fatigue during long working hours. Patients- anesthetist relationship, helping them, answering all patients questions, managing all their complaints, preoperative care includes reassurance, assessment. Good intraoperative management includes monitoring, adjust drug doses .postoperative care includes, and pain management care and hemodynamic parameter. In this book there are simple guides for good safe anesthesia. I wrote this book as simple points to be easy, quick revision of all important items must be satisfied to allow good safe anesthesia.

Simple guides for good anesthetist:

Skills and practice

1. knowledge of the law and other regulation relevant to their practice
2. stick on to the laws and codes of practice related to their work
3. Keep knowledge and skills up to date.
4. New improved techniques for patient wellbeing and safety to be acquired.
5. Contribute in qualified progress and learning activities.
6. Create a personal advance plan.
7. Attend hospital and departmental educational meetings.
8. Look for facilitates to learn from colleagues locally and somewhere else.
9. Keep records of CPD activities to support the revalidation process.
10. Take part in regular and systematic audit.
11. The Good Anaesthetist will be made available online as a web based resource.
12. Regular evaluation personal practice at regular intervals.
13. When a difficulty arises outside their area of skill calling help from a suitable colleague
14. Assume different approaches to learning and teaching.
15. Work within the limits of their skill; and where suitable consult or try to find advice from other sources or refer patients to colleagues, including those from other specialties,.
16. Skills, attitudes and practice of a competent teacher/trainer, must be applied.
17. Share in the assessment of trainees, having undertaken the required training.

Anesthetist health:

Anesthetist fitness is important, chronic diseases, as hypertension, diabetes, pregnancy.

Stress fatigue, addiction, mental problems.

Common health worker transmitted diseases, in hospital, during preoperative patient's assessments, intraoperative blood born transmitted diseases.

1. Regular medical assessment for anesthetist, guidance if he knows that anesthetist may have a serious condition which either could affect anesthetist performance or is transmissible to patients.
2. When there is mental health problem, including addiction, which could potentially affect their professional judgment or performance, anesthetist should access professional counseling, advice, support and help services
3. protect patients and colleagues from their own health or other problem.
4. Immunization against common serious communicable diseases where vaccines are available. Hepatitis B vaccine, meningitis, influenza, measles, mumps, rubella, and varicella.
5. Those for which active and/or passive immunization of HCWs may be indicated in certain circumstances (i.e., tuberculosis, hepatitis A, meningococcal disease, typhoid fever, and vaccinia) or in the future (i.e., pertussis).
6. Those for which immunization of all adults is recommended (i.e., tetanus, diphtheria, and pneumococcal disease).
7. Help colleague if judgment or ability is temporarily impaired due to stress, tiredness or illness.
8. Avoidance work under the influence of alcohol or drugs.
9. A healthy anesthetist is one who can contribute fully to a team and, in turn, the effective provision of medical care

safety and quality

1. Report risks in the healthcare environment to their employing or contracting bodies.
2. Ensure that there is continuous supervision of a patient receiving anesthesia. If in exceptional circumstances you are required to leave the theatre, you must ensure that the patient is supervised by another anesthetist or appropriately trained assistant
3. Respond promptly to risks posed by patients.
4. Follow infection control procedures and regulations. and protect the health and well being of vulnerable people, including children and the elderly and those with learning disabilities.
5. Must take action where there is evidence that a colleague's conduct, performance or health may be putting patients at risk.
6. Listen impartially to medical, nursing and other colleagues when they express concerns about a fellow anesthetist
7. Responsibilities in regard to occupational health and safety laws apply to all employees in an organization, and discuss such concerns only in an appropriate forum.
8. Participate in relevant national reporting schemes.
9. support legitimate requests for information from organizations monitoring public health.
10. Provide information for confidential enquiries and significant event reporting.
11. Report suspected adverse drug reactions, or in active anesthesia drugs .
12. Guarantee that on-call teams have a range of skills sufficient to manage any reasonable predictable clinical contingency.
13. Write clear instructions for post-operative care including pain relief, oxygen therapy and fluid management, monitoring of postoperative bleeding.
14. Ensure that recovering patients are observed on a one-to-one basis by an anesthetist, recovery nurse or other properly trained member of staff .
15. Child protection and the anesthetist: safeguarding children in the operating theatre.

16. Anesthesia and peri-operative care of the elderly.

17. Act quickly and suitably when anesthetic complications arise and are familiar with the operation of resuscitation equipment and current resuscitation guidelines.

18. Take urgent appropriate action if a patient has suffered hurt through accident or for any other reason.

19. An anesthetist must use safe, regularly maintained equipment which has been checked before use, and use equipment and techniques with which he or she is familiar.

20. Adequately assess the patient's condition.

21. An anaesthetist must assess the patient before anesthesia and devise an appropriate plan of anesthetic management.

22. An anesthetist must provide or arrange advice, investigations or treatment where necessary.

23. An anesthetist must prescribe drugs or treatment, including repeat prescriptions, safely and appropriately.

24. An anaesthetist must take steps to alleviate pain and distress whether or not a cure may be possible. ❏

25. An anaesthetist must provide effective treatments based on the best available evidence.

26. Consider appropriate local or nationally agreed guidelines when planning an anaesthetic.

27. An anaesthetist must consult colleagues, or refer patients to colleagues, when this is in the patient's best interest.

Basic Anesthesia Machine Set-Up Checklist

Prior to Setting up Anesthesia Machine

- Turn oxygen ON, if pressure is at or below 500 pounds per square inch it is time to open a second tank
- Turn alarm ON
- Turn scavenger ON

Basic Anesthesia Machine Set-Up

- All anesthesia machines vary, so know your machine
- All parts of the machine must be wiped down with a disinfectant
- Touch and tighten all fittings on machine
- Make sure pop-off valve is in the open position
- Attach breathing hose with Y connector or nonrebreathing system (depending on weight of first surgical patient)
- Attach reservoir bag (depending on the weight of the first surgical patient)
- Check/fill anesthetic in vaporizer
- Check and change carbon dioxide granules or F/Air canister prn
- Attach exhaust hose from anesthesia machine to exhaust outlet

Pressurize Anesthesia Machine

- Close pop-off valve
- Occlude end of breathing tube with your thumb
- Quickly push oxygen flush button to fill bag
- Look at the pressure gauge, the pressure should hold steady if there are no leaks
- With the other hand gently press on the reservoir bag and hold the pressure on the gauge for 45 seconds. If there is no drop in pressure, your machine is leak-free.
- If the pressure held, turn off oxygen, open pop-off valve, and the machine and the bag you tested it with are ready
- Test each reservoir bag prior to first use of the day
- If the pressure does not hold, you need to look further for a leak prior to using the machine

Checking For a Leak in the Anesthesia Machine

- Get a spray bottle of soapy water and a hand towel
- Close pop-off valve

- Occlude end of breathing tube with your thumb
- Turn oxygen up to 1 liter
- Fill anesthesia bag
- Using the spray bottle, spray one area of the machine at a time, gently press on the reservoir bag and watch for bubbles to form on the machine. Also listen; you may hear the leak before you see it. Key areas are the bag neck, site of hose connection to machine, and the soda sorb canister where it connects to machine.
- Once the leak is found, dry the area, repair the problem, spray with water and check to be sure the leak is truly fixed. Repeat pressurizing the machine.
- If no leak has yet to be found continue to another part of the anesthesia machine following the above procedure until the leak is found and the machine is 100% functioning.
- Record on a log form (see our Specialty Folder for an example of this form)

Safe anesthesia during radiologic investigations

- General, anesthesia and sedation are safe for most patients.
- Patients are closely monitored under the direct, continuous care of an anesthesiologist or non-anesthesiologist, regardless of the level of sedation or anesthesia they have received.
- Serious side effects and allergic reactions resulting from anesthesia are rare.
- Common complications following sedation or general anesthesia include nausea, vomiting, dizziness, headache, sore throat, blood pressure changes and pain. These side effects are usually mild, short-lived and sometimes treatable with medication.
- Some patients, both adults and children, may not achieve adequate sedation and pain relief with sedative administration and may require a procedure to be rescheduled with general anesthesia.
- More serious complications from anesthesia are rare and are more likely to occur in patients with complex, serious medical conditions.

Monitoring:

Monitoring equipment, machines for delivery of anesthetic gases, ventilators that function for preterm infants through adults, and intravenous infusion pumps are now routinely used in the MR suite. This equipment must meet three criteria:

1. pose no danger to the patient either by spontaneous movement within the magnetic field or overheating
2. have no effect on procuring good images (ferrous metal next to the anatomic area being scanned will distort the image)
3. function properly within the magnetic field (no torque on ferromagnetic circuitry).These goals can be achieved by keeping ferromagnetic equipment outside of the gauss line, by replacing ferromagnetic parts in conventional equipment with aluminum or plastic, or by purchasing equipment and monitors specifically created (and FDA approved) for use in the MR suite.

Systems for central wall gases (oxygen, air and nitrous oxide) are commercially available and can be installed during construction of the MR suite

Suction (both for patient care and evacuation of gases)

Electrical power sources consisting of isolated duplex power circuits with filtered 120V

Oxygenation

- pulse oximeters function well in the magnet, severe burns to extremities have been caused by the induction of current within a loop of wire. This may be avoided by placing the sensor on the extremity distal to the magnet, oximeters use heavy fiberoptic cables,
- The magnet superconductors are kept cool in liquid nitrogen. , the ambient oxygen supply of the room can drop precipitously, causing hypoxia and the potential for cryo injury. Quench monitors within each MRI suite recognize changes in room oxygen concentration.

Scanned respiratory capnography direct visualization of the airway may be possible

Electrocardiographic monitoring is

- Maximum voltage charges are induced in any column of conducting fluid (blood within the transverse aorta) when the fluid flow is 90 degrees to the field (supine patient in MR scanner).
- Plethysmography (as seen in the oximetry waveform) can be used as a heart tachometer, but is not useful for ischemia or arrhythmia detection.
- 12-lead ECG pre- and post, In patients highly susceptible to ischemia, a utilizing ECG electrodes made of carbon graphite to lower resistance, eliminate ferromagnetism, and minimize RF interference.

Oscillo metric blood pressure monitoring

MR-approved monitoring systems use automated, which, because it is based on pneumatic principles, avoids electromagnetic interference

Temperature

During MRI, body temperature may increase from heating caused by RF within the magnetic field or decrease from the cool environment necessary to protect superconductors.

Thermistors to monitor temperature are not practical because of the ferromagnetic content of the cables. Liquid crystal thermometers may be used, although their accuracy is limited. Anesthesia

Ventilation:

- Because of the magnet depth, nearly 2m, it is often virtually impossible to visualize the patient's face and chest for adequacy of ventilation during scanning. Noise levels of 95 decibels-equivalent to light road work-are frequently appreciated in 1.5 T scanners, making auscultation of the lungs during scanning almost impossible. (Ear plugs are recommended for anesthetized or sedated patients for noise protection.)

- Anesthesia machines can be modified for use in a magnetic field by replacing. Currently, manufacturers offer MRI-compatible machines made largely of stainless steel, brass, aluminum and plastic.

- Regardless of the mode of anesthetic and for critical care patients, mechanical ventilation may be required.
- Plastic battery-operated laryngoscopes may be used for tracheal intubation.
- Batteries will last longer if shielded with a paper casing or plastic coating. Conversely, the airway can be secured using conventional laryngoscopes before the patient is moved into the scanner.
- Only medical gas cylinders constructed from aluminum should be used in the MRI suite.

Anesthesiologist patient relation ship

1. Keep patients informed about the progress of their care.
An anesthetist must listen to patients and respect their views about their health.
2. Give patients the information they need in order to make decisions about their care in a way they can understand.
3. Encourage questions when possible and allow time to listen to the concerns of patients, guardians or parents before and, where possible, after an anaesthetic or therapeutic procedure.
4. Give patients the information they need in order to make decisions about their care in a way they can understand.
5. Encourage questions when possible and allow time to listen to the concerns of patients, guardians or parents before and, where possible, after an anaesthetic or therapeutic procedure.
6. Respond to patients' questions.
7. Answer questions openly and honestly. communicate effectively
8. Should encourage patients to take an interest in their health and take action to improve and maintain it.
9. Support patients in caring for themselves.
10. Educate patients about different methods for pain relief, PCR, epidural analgesia .Verbal information, Written and/or audiovisual information Brochures, Wall posters, Video films Web pages.

11. Document pain regularly, take appropriate action and monitor efficacy and side effects of treatment.
12. Record the information in a well-defined place in the patient record, such as the vital sign sheet or a purposed signed acute pain chart.
13. The nurse responsible for the patient reports the intensity of pain and treats the pain within the defined rules of the local guidelines.
14. The physician responsible for the patient may need to modify the intervention if evaluation shows that the patient still has significant pain.

15. Engage in the education of patients and the wider public.
16. Satisfied that they have consent or other valid authority before they undertake any examination or investigation, provide treatment or involve patients in teaching or research.
17. ensure that patients have understood the nature and purpose of any proposed treatment or investigation and any significant risk or side effects associated with it, enabling them to make an informed choice of anaesthetic technique by giving clear explanation of the advantages and disadvantages of the options available, using terms that a patient can understand and relate to when giving consent.
18. Must abide with local research ethics committee and multicentre research ethics committee guidelines when carrying out research.
19. Anesthetist must maintain patient confidentiality at all times.
20. Be polite, considerate and honest and respect patients' dignity and privacy.
21. Promote trust with patients through courteous behavior, honest discussions and respect for their right to privacy and dignity, whether conscious or unconscious.
22. Treat each patient fairly and as an individual.
23. Respond constructively to any complaints received and cooperate with any relevant complaints procedures or formal inquiry into the treatment of a patient.
24. Provide care on the basis of the patient's needs and the likely effect of treatment.
25. Act in the patient's interest at all times.

26. Must not allow their personal prejudice to affect the treatment or management of a patient under their care.

Anesthesia team work

Members of the Anesthesia Care Team work together to provide the optimal anesthesia experience for all patients.

Core members of the anesthesia care team include

- Both physicians (anesthesiologist, anesthesiology fellow, anesthesiology resident),

- nonphysicians (anesthesiologist assistant, nurse anesthetist, anesthesiologist assistant student, student nurse anesthetist).

- Other health care professionals also make important contributions to the perianesthetic care of the patient.

Aim of anesthesia team To provide optimum patient safety.

The anesthesiologist directing the Anesthesia Care Team is responsible for management of team personnel, patient pre-anesthetic evaluation, prescribing the anesthetic plan, management of the anesthetic, post-anesthesia care and anesthesia consultation.

1. Communicate clearly and effectively with colleagues within and outside the team.
2. Pass on information to colleagues involved in, or taking over, the care of your patient.
3. Communicate directly with senior and specialist medical colleagues when appropriate.
4. Communicate effectively with all members of the team to ensure resources are used to best effect for the delivery of patient care.
5. explain to assistants and other staff what your requirements are likely to be in advance of inducing anesthesia
6. Treat colleagues fairly and with respect.
7. Respect the skills and contributions of other members of the anaesthetic, medical and nursing team.

14

8.   Encourage multidisciplinary team working.

9.   Ensure that the work content of job plans and on-call rotas is fairly distributed among colleagues.

10. Support colleagues who have problems with their performance, conduct or health.

11. Be willing to advise and help colleagues.

12. Support colleagues undergoing rehabilitation after their illness or returning to work after a period of absence for any reason.

13. Act as a positive role model for colleagues.

14. Provide appropriate professional support and encouragement for trainees, staff and associate specialist grade (SAS) doctors and other anesthetists under their supervision.

15. Attend hospital rapidly when requested and only leave when appropriate to do so.

16. Prepare to work smoothly within the department.

17. Ensure that they are aware of being placed on a schedule to cover emergency operating lists and on-call duties.

18. Make sure that when on-call they can easily be contacted.

19. Arrange annual, professional and study leave in advance in accordance with local departmental policy.

20. Ensure that colleagues to whom they delegate have appropriate qualifications and experience.

21. Must not exaggerate competence or fail to mention significant weaknesses in a reference.

22. Be honest and open in relations with colleagues.

23. Provide references, reports or signed documents within a reasonable time.

24. Make sure that an applicant is aware that a reservation would be expressed when writing a reference for him or her.

25. Respond rapidly and fully to complaints.

26. Give an explanation to the patient and their relatives and explain in understandable terms what occurred when an untoward incident took place.

27. Consider the clinical needs of the patient and the professional needs of colleagues when planning a clinical session.

28. Deal with your colleagues fairly and without discrimination, irrespective of their gender, age, race, sexuality, economic status, lifestyle, culture and religious or political belief, is essential when working as part of a team.

29. Consideration of a colleague's competence and performance must be based on honest and objective decisions and judgments. Honesty and objectivity must also be applied in your professional relationships with patients.

30. Best practice involves the recognition and acknowledgement of different needs in helping patients access medical care on an equal basis

31. Complaints must also be managed fairly and without discrimination.

career and financial aspects of anesthesiologist:

1. support the specialty of anesthesia in the wider public interest

2. Make sure that they have adequate indemnity or insurance cover for their practice.

3. Be honest in financial and commercial dealings.
   Inform patients about any fees and charges before starting treatment.

4. Ensure any published information about their services is factual and verifiable.

5. Should not undertake private practice or any other commitment which would prevent them from fulfilling scheduled clinical NHS duties.

6. t be honest in any formal statement or report, whether written or oral, making clear the limits of your knowledge or competence.

7. Divergence away from these virtues, regardless of where an anesthetist may be working (e.g. the NHS or private healthcare sector), risks diminishing the trust placed in anesthetists and the profession by patients, colleagues and the public.

8. In providing information about yourself, your services and others, honesty is reflected by the accuracy and verifiability of that information. Fulfilling contractual and professional obligations to their employer and patients will demonstrate the integrity of an anesthetist.

Preoperative preparation:

    a. Patient assessment.

- **Aims of the preoperative patient assessment**

- Establish a doctor patient relationship.

- recognize medical problems required more management.

- Risk assessment of anesthesia and surgery.

- To compare preoperative vital signs with intra and postoperative proceedings.

- Obtain an informed consent from the patient.

How to assess patients

(A) History taking

(B) Physical examination.

(C) Investigations.

(D) Risk assessment.

(A) History taking.

Patient's personal data

- Name, age, body weight, and ASA physical status.

- Scheduled operation: Diagnosis, site, and side. .

Medical history

- Present and past surgical and medical history and hospitalizations.

- Previous unfavorable anesthesia history:

Difficult endotracheal intubation,

Exposure to Halothane anesthesia within 6 months,

Delayed recovery.

- Family history of anesthesia:

Succinylcholine apnea.

- Female of child-bearing age: early pregnancy as anaesthetic agents may be teratogenic and induce abortion.
- Late pregnancy there is an increased risk of aspiration of gastric contents and premature labour).
- Contraceptive pills (DVT).

History Special habits

- Cigarette Smoking.
- Drug abuse.
- Alcohol.

Drug history:

Current medications, allergies, and drug interactions between

Anaesthetic agents and antihypertensive and antidepressant drugs.

(B) Physical examination

- Genera! Examination: Vital signs, base line mental status, evaluation of heart and lungs, and abdominal examination, lower limb edema

Airway assessment

The aim is to prepare algorithm of difficult intubation.

Patient scheduled for regional anesthesia:

- History of anticoagulant drugs,
- anatomical landmarks', and
- Detect contraindication for regional anesthesia.
- If there was any adverse effect after previous regional.

(C) Investigations

- CBC, coagulation profile, fasting blood sugar, renal and liver functions.
- Chest x-ray and ECG for patient above 50 years or if indicated. . Special tests if indicated; as echocardiography.

(D) Risk assessment:

American Society of Anesthesiologists (ASA) physical status classification is a scale used io assess patient's general physical status

- ASA 1: Fit and healthy patient.
- ASA 2: Patient with mild controlled systemic disease not limiting normal activity. e.g. Controlled hypertension.
- ASA 3: Patient with moderate systemic disease limiting normal activity, e.g. Renal failure,
- ASA 4: Patient with severe systemic disease that is a constant threat to life. e.g. Acute myocardial infarction.
- ASA 5: A morbid patient not expected to survive 24 hours, e.g. Ruptured abdominal aortic aneurysm in shock.
- (ASA 6) emergency procedure. A brain dead patient is usually designated

(E) Patient preparation

- manage un controlled conditions as hypertension, un controlled blood glucose.

- STOP smoking for 24 hours reduces intra and .

- Obtain an informed consent for anaesthesia , surgery and informed label over the patient's wrist (patient's name and operation site). '*.

- Remove all cosmetics, dentures, contact lens, and prostneses.

- Empty the bladder.

- Prepare for blood and/or its components according to the operation type and the patient's preoperative condition.

preoperative fasting:

Aim of preoperative fasting to decrease the incidence of regurgitation and pulmonary aspiration of gastric contents

Risk of pulmonary regurgitation:

- Recent food intake,
- Opioids,
- Abdominal distention (obesity, pregnancy, and ascites).
- altered gastrointestinal motility,
- emergency surgery,
- trauma,
- diabetes mellitus
- Renal failure.

Duration of fasting:

- 2 hours after clear liquids (20ml of water for oral medications).

- 4 hours after breast milk for pediatric patients.
- 6 hours after light meals.
- 8 hours after fatty and meat foods. Chest x-ray of aspiration
- 12 hours for cs operation.
- Fasting after midnight for morning operation, clear liquid 20ml up to 2 hours before afternoon operation.
- fasting for 6 hours if possible for emergency operation

<u>**preoperative medications:**</u>

- Continue most chronic drug therapy until operation morning except anticoagulants, diabetes and digitalis medications.
- Oral benzodiazepine the night before the operation.
- Metoclopramide, Ranitidine, Sodium Citrate for palient at risk of aspiration,
- - Morning dose of current medications as antihypertensives.
- 2. Benzodiazepine
- . Midazolam and Diazepam.
- • Relief anxiety, sedation, and ante grade amnesia. .
- The main indication for premedication.
- Opioid
- Morphine and Pethidine.
- Enhance smooth induction and maintenance of anesthesia and reduce the required postopcrative analgesia (Preemptive analgesia).
- Anticholinergic agents . Atropine.
  Reduce airways secretion and prevent reflex Brady cardia.
- Antiemetic, H_2 blockers, Antacids, and Proton pump inhibitors. Metoclopramide, Ranitidine, Sodium Citrate, and Omeprazole, Accelerate gastric emptying, reduce volume and acidity of gastric content prophylaxis against aspiration, and reduce postoperative nausea and vomiting.
- Antibiotic prophylaxis for patients at risk of infective endocarditic blood viscosity, platelet postoperative respiratory

Preoperative patient visit:

- Reassurances by Visit the patient the day before the operation explain operation, and post operative pain control.

preoperative consent

- Informed consent must be taken from all patients
- If the patients are not competent to consent, a legal guardian must singe the consent. .
- Consent is not necessary for life saving procedure and for unconscious patient.
- Possible risks and alternatives to the procedure.

when to postpone elective operation:

- Chronic diseases are not under optimum control.
- Acute upper respiratory tract infection.
- Recent food intake,
- Refusal to sign the informed consent.
- Pregnancy.

When to postpone emergency operation:

Postpone emergency operations without adequate resuscitation unless there is extensive and/or continuous bleeding and life threatens problem.

Cigarette Smoking and anesthesia:

- Cigarette smoke contains CO which increases CO Hb level (Up to 15% of the Hb) and decreases arterial 0_2 content.
- COHb ti« is short 4-6 hrs.
- Nicotine increases the myocardial 62 consumption aggregation, ischemic heart disease,   COPD, complications and risk of malignancy.

- Smoking increases intra and postoperative morbidity.

- Advantage of preoperative cessation of smoking:

- 1 2 hours: Decrease COHb level and decrease coronary vascular resistance. Increase arterial 0; content.

- 2 days: Abolish nicotine stimulant effect on CVS and improve cilliary function.

- 2 weeks: Decrease sputum volume to normal level.

- 2 months: Decrease chronic bronchitis (bronchospasm and secretions).

Immune system and liver enzymes return to normal. NB: Informed consent for anesthesia and surgery.

Prophylaxis against deep venous thrombosis(DVT)

DVT that starts in the venous plexuses of the lower limb ,and pelvis ,and extends up into the femoral and iliac veins. PE usually results from (DVT) is responsible for 10% of all hospital deaths. PE usually happens after 3-21days of operation.

High risk patients for DVT:

- Prolonged bed   rest.
- Pregnancy.
- Puerperium.
- Estrogen.
- Obesity.
- Old age.
- Dehydration
- Hypercoagulability state
- Trauma, and cancer.
- Progestogen contraceptive don't increase risk of DVT.

Prophylaxis against DVT:

1. Prophylactic anticoagulants: Heparin 5000units SC/12hours reduces incidence of DVT and PE.

2. Warfarin and Aspirin provide some protection against venous thromboembolism.

3. Compression stockings and pneumatic leg compression devices during operation.

4. Early mobilization, breathing exercise, avoid prolonged bed rest and dehydration.

Treatment of DVT:

Analgesia, treat dysrhythmia, starts Heparin, and surgery.

preoperative check list:

Preoperative Anesthesia Machine Checklist Recommendations

In 2008, the ASA, along with the American Association of Nurse Anesthetists (AANA) and the American Academy of Anesthesiologists Assistants (AAAA), endorsed updated general recommendations for the daily and pre-procedural checks of the modern anesthesia machine or work station, which appear on the ASA website along with sample check lists for particular machines developed by the hospitals across the country. These general recommendations are summarized as:

TO BE COMPLETED DAILY

	Item to Be Completed	**Responsible Party**
1	Verify Auxiliary Oxygen Cylinder and Self-inflating Manual Ventilation Device are Available & Functioning	Provider and Tech
2	Verify patient suction is adequate to clear the airway	Provider and Tech
3	Turn on anesthesia delivery system and confirm that ac power is available	Provider or Tech
4	Verify availability of required monitors, including alarms	Provider or Tech
5	Verify that pressure is adequate on the spare oxygen cylinder mounted on the anesthesia machine	Provider and Tech
6	Verify that the piped gas pressures are ≥ 50 psig	Provider and Tech
7	Verify that vaporizers are adequately filled and, if applicable, that the filler ports are tightly closed	Provider or Tech
8	Verify that there are no leaks in the gas supply lines between the flowmeters and the common gas outlet	Provider or Tech
9	Test scavenging system function	Provider or Tech
10	Calibrate, or verify calibration of, the oxygen monitor and check	Provider or Tech

the low oxygen alarm

11	Verify carbon dioxide absorbent is not exhausted	Provider or Tech
12	Breathing system pressure and leak testing	Provider and Tech
13	Verify that gas flows properly through the breathing circuit during both inspiration and exhalation	Provider and Tech
14	Document completion of checkout procedures	Provider and Tech
15	Confirm ventilator settings and evaluate readiness to deliver anesthesia care (ANESTHESIA TIME OUT)	Provider

TO BE COMPLETED PRIOR TO EACH PROCEDURE

	Item to Be Completed	Responsible Party
2	Verify patient suction is adequate to clear the airway	Provider and Tech
4	Verify availability of required monitors, including alarms	Provider or Tech
7	Verify that vaporizers are adequately filled and if applicable that the filler ports are tightly closed.	Provider
11	Verify carbon dioxide absorbent is not exhausted	Provider or Tech
12	Breathing system pressure and leak testing	Provider and Tech
13	Verify that gas flows properly through the breathing circuit during both inspiration and exhalation	Provider and Tech
14	Document completion of checkout procedures	Provider and Tech
15	Confirm ventilator settings and evaluate readiness to deliver anesthesia care (ANESTHESIA TIME OUT)	

Pacemaker and implantable cardioverter defibrillator

This practice advisory provides evidence-based recommendations on the preoperative evaluation, preoperative preparation and reprogramming, intraoperative management, and necessary postoperative management for patients with pacemakers and internal cardioverter-defibrillators, as well as patients with devices designed to provide the newer cardiac resynchronization therapy.

This guideline is revised slightly from the last version published in 2005. It has useful recommendations for management of these implanted electronic devices during multiple types of specialized surgical procedures. It is based primarily on the small amount of evidence currently available, and so its recommendations are somewhat limited

Monitoring:

Continuous evaluation of the patient's oxygenation, ventilation temperature, using clinical sense and monitoring equipment .

Timing of monitoring:

Monitoring should be started before induction and continued full recovery from anesthesia.

Cardiovascular monitoring

- o Palpation of the pulse and auscultation of the heart sounds.
- o   BP and heart rate monitored and evaluated at least every 5 minutes.
- o Non invasive measurement of the ABP: Manually or automated.
- o Invasive (direct) measurement: An arterial cannula is placed in an artery (usually radial artery) and connected to a fluid filled tube to a pressure transducer It is an accurate measurement used for major operation, haemodynamically unstable patient, induced controlled hypotension, and for frequent arterial blood sampling. Complications: thrombosis, infection, and bleeding.
- o MAP = DBP + 1/3 Pulse pressure (SBP-DBP).
- o ECG Monitor heart rate, rhythm, myocardial ischaemia, electrolytes abnormalities, and pace maker.

o ECG does not monitor the myocardial mechanical function and the COP.

o If ECG confirms VT deliver a DC shock.

o If ECG confirms asystole, give Adrenaline and consider Atropine.

o Heart rhythms associated with cardiac arrest include: VF, pulse less ventricular tachycardia, pulse less electrical activity, and asystole.

(B) Ventilation monitoring:

Pulse oximetry: Device used for continuous non invasive monitoring of arterial O2 saturation and heart rate. Normal range is 100%-97%.

- Detects hypoxaemia early before cyanosis appears. .

Capnography: Device used for continuous non invasive monitoring of End-tidal C02 concentration.

- Normal range: 35 - 45 mmHg.

- Assess adequacy of ventilation.

- Confirm endotracheal intubation.

- Detect pulmonary embolism.

(C) Body temperature monitoring:

Hypothermia is a core body temperature < 35 °C. Hypothermia is a common cause of delayed recovery from anesthesia especially in infant and elderly patients. Temperature must be monitored when significant changes in temperature are intended or suspected.

Thermistor: Device used for monitoring core body temperature by a probe which is placed in nasopharynx, oesophagus, or rectum.

. Prevention and treatment of hypothermia: Cover all unused exposed body surfaces. Warm water blanket and forced warm air blanket. Warm all transfused fluids, blood products, and irrigation solutions.

(D) Neuromuscular transmission monitoring Peripheral Nerve stimulator: Device used to assess degree of neuromuscular blockade by stimulating a motor nerve and evaluating muscle contractions

1. during general anesthesia

- Measure degree of muscle relaxation and detect time for the next dose of muscles relaxant during surgery .it Measures degree of reversal of neuromuscular blockade before endotracheal extubation.

2. during regional anesthesia: Locates the proper anatomical site of a nerve to be blocked.

Intraoperative fluid management:

Fluid therapy Healthy adult can balance daily fluid input and output (about 2.5L water/day/70 kg).

- Estimated blood volume (ml/kg body weight):

- Fluid Distribution in 70 kg adult according to "60, 40, and 20" rule:

Manifestation of preoperative fluid deficit:

- Dry mouth
- Thirst.
- Decreased skin turgor,
- drowsiness,
- Oliguria, Orthostatic hypotension,
- Tachycardia,
- Tachypnoea,
- cool extremities,
- Metabolic acidosis.

Monitoring Intraoperative of fluid replacement

- BP, HR,
- urine out (1ml/kg/hr),
- CVP (5-10cm H2O)

- Intraoperative fluid replacement.

  - Basal hourly requirement + Preoperative fiuid deficits + Operative fluid loss.
    - Rate of fluid replacement: 1^{5i} hr gives 50%, 2nd hr give 25%, and $3'''$ hr give 25%.

(D)<u>Blood and blood products</u>: Each whole blood unit contains 350-400 ml; one blood unit increases the haematocrit level by 3% and Hb level by 1 gm/dt.

Fresh frozen plasma and cryoprecipitate must be ABO compatible.

Platelets transfusion indicatations:

Probably the most controversial threshold is for the clinically stable patient with an intact vascular system and normal platelet function. Prophylactic platelet transfusions may be appropriate at 5,000- 10,000/uL to prevent spontaneous bleeding. Patients with autoimmune destruction of platelets, such as ITP, may not receive therapeutic benefit from prophylactic transfusion, but may however benefit from transfusion if bleeding.

- thrombocytopenia
- platelet dysfunction
- treat active platelet-related bleeding
- Prophylaxis in those at serious risk of bleeding.
- myelodysplasia, aplastic anemia,
- solid tumors,
- congenital or acquired/medication-induced platelet dysfunction,
- Central nervous system trauma.
- patients undergoing extracorporeal membrane oxygenation
- cardiopulmonary bypass may also need platelet transfusion.

Dosing of platelets transfusion:

- Typical dosing for an adult is a pool of 6 whole blood derived (sometimes referred to as random donor) platelets or one apheresis platelet. This is expected to raise the platelet count by 30,000-60,000/uL in a 70 kg patient.
- Transfused platelets have a short life span and will need to be re-dosed within 3-4 days if given for prophylaxis.

- Suboptimal increases can be seen due to non-immune destruction or immune refractoriness. If suboptimal increases are suspected, the corrected count increment (CCI) can help determine if the response is truly suboptimal based on amount of platelets transfused compared to body surface area. The CCI can also assist in determining whether the response is due to immune refractoriness or non-immune causes.
- Thresholds for transfusion due to thrombocytopenia have been controversial. However it is generally accepted that a count of 50,000/uL is sufficient for most invasive procedures including most surgeries.
- Platelet counts of >100,000/uL are recommended for ophthalmic ,and neurosurgery. Higher transfusion thresholds may be appropriate for patients with platelet dysfunction.

.

Intra operative special anesthesia techniques:

Hypotensive anesthesia:

Aim of Hypotensive anesthesia:

- controlled hypotension has been used to reduce bleeding and the need for blood transfusions,
- provide a satisfactory bloodless surgical field

indication of Hypotensive anesthesia

- oromaxillofacial surgery (mandibular osteotomy, facial repair),
- endoscopic sinus or middle ear microsurgery,
- spinal surgery and other neurosurgery (aneurysm),
- major orthopaedic surgery (hip or knee replacement, spinal),
- prostatectomy, cardiovascular surgery and liver transplant surgery.
- Controlled hypotension is defined as a reduction of the systolic blood pressure to 80-90 mm Hg, a reduction of mean arterial pressure (MAP) to 50-65 mm Hg or a 30% reduction of baseline MAP.

Pharmacological agents used for controlled hypotension :

- New drugs and techniques have been recently evaluated for their ability to induce effective hypotension without impairing the perfusion of vital organs.
- This development has been aided by new knowledge on the physiology of peripheral microcirculatory regulation.
- Apart from the adverse effects of major hypotension on the perfusion of vital organs, potent hypotensive agents have their own adverse effects depending on their concentration, which can be reduced by adjuvant treatment.
- Care with use limits the major risks of these agents in controlled hypotension; risks that are generally less important than those of transfusion or alternatives to transfusion.

Criteria of good Hypotensive agents

- It must be easy to administer,
- have a short onset time, an effect that disappears quickly when administration is discontinued,
- a rapid elimination without toxic metabolites,
- Negligible effects on vital organs, and a predictable and dose-dependent effect.
- Inhalation agents (isoflurane, sevoflurane) provide the benefit of being hypnotic and hypotensive agents at clinical concentrations, and are used alone or in combination with adjuvant agents to limit tachycardia and rebound hypertension, for example, inhibitors of the autonomic nervous system (clonidine, beta-blockers) or ACE inhibitors.
- When they are used alone, inhalation anaesthetics require high concentrations for a significant reduction in bleeding that can lead to hepatic or renal injury.
- The greatest efficacy and ease-of-use to toxicity ratio is for techniques of anesthesia that associate analgesia and hypotension at clinical concentrations without the need for potent hypotensive agents.
- Drugs that can be used successfully alone and those that are used adjunctively to limit dosage requirements and, therefore, the adverse effects of the other agents.

- Drugs used successfully alone include inhalation anaesthetics, sodium nitroprusside, nitroglycerin, trimethaphan camsilate, alprostadil (prostaglandin E1), adenosine, remifentanil, and agents used in spinal anaesthesia.
- Drugs that can be used alone or in combination include calcium channel antagonists (e.g. nicardipine), beta-adrenoceptor antagonists (beta-blockers) [e.g. propranolol, esmolol] and Fenoldopam
- Drugs that are mainly used adjunctively include ACE inhibitors and clonidine.
- New hypotensive drugs, such as fenoldopam, adenosine and alprostadil, are currently being evaluated; however, they have disadvantages and a high treatment cost that limits their development in this indication.
- New techniques of controlled hypotension subscribe to the use of the natural hypotensive effect of the anaesthetic drug with regard to the definition of the ideal hypotensive agent.

The first and oldest technique is epidural anaesthesia, but depending on the surgery, it is not always appropriate. The most recent satisfactory technique is a combination treatment of remifentanil with either propofol or an inhalation agent (isoflurane, desflurane or sevoflurane) at clinical concentrations.

Ultrasonographic nerve blochade:

The main advantages are:

- It allows even the less skilled anesthetist to use it.
- Training may take very short time compared with other techniques.
- It allows injection of the local anesthestic in a proper time.
- it decreases the incidence of complication during peripheral nerve blockade as intravascular or intraneural injection.

Knobology:

Knowledge of basic applied ultrasound physics, it is Major skill categories Learning objectives Operation of the ultrasound machine.

The anesthetist must know

1-how to capture and archive images and video loops Image optimization.

2-Appropriate probe and frequency selection

3- How to adjust and optimize important machine settings, e.g. depth, focus, gain Image

4- Cross-sectional anatomy.

5- Recognition of sonographic appearance of relevant structures (nerves, vessels, bone, pleura, peritoneum).

7- Plane and out-of-plane needle approaches, and their benefits and limitations Probe handling skills pressure, basic movements of alignment, rotation and tilting.

8-organization of probe and needle in the in-plane and out-of-plane approaches..

9- Unsuitable needle location, e.g. intramuscular

10-Recognition of appropriate local anesthetic spread

Preparation and check list for peripheral nerve blockade:

Intravenous accesses is mandatory.

Monitoring:

Aim of close monitoring.

Local anesthestic toxicity

It is biphasic it may be immediately or during injection or 10-30 minutes after injection.sign of toxicity after intravascular injection 1-2 minutes and after absorbtion of local anesthesitic 10-30.

Monitoring:

1. Pulse oximetry
2. Noninvasive blood pressure
3. Electrocardiogram
4. Respiratory rate
5. Mental status

Emergency drugs must be presented:

Drug	Suggested Dose (70 Kg Adult)
Atropine	**0.2 mg - 0.4 mg IV increments**
Ephedrine	5 mg - 10 mg IV
Phenylephrine	50 µg - 200 µg IV
Epinephrine	10 µg - 100 µg IV
Midazolam	2.0 mg - 10 mg IV
Propofol*	30 mg - 200 mg IV
Muscle relaxant (succinylcholine)	Succinylcholine: 20 - 80 mg IV
Intralipid 20%	105 mL IV bolus followed by 0.25 mL/kg/min infusion given at rate of 400 mL over 10 min

Emergency ventilation equipments :

- Oxygenation.
- Intubation.
- Ventilator.
- Help.

Skills needed for cardiothoracic anesthesia:

According to cardiothoracic anesthesiology one month dedicated to transesophageal echocardiography, one month in cardiothoracic intensive care unit and two months of elective rotation which includes inpatient or outpatient cardiology or pulmonary medicine, invasive cardiology, medical or surgical critical care and extracorporeal perfusion technology.

neuroprotection, myocardial protection, blood conservation strategies, and port access surgery.

Anesthesiologist and CPR:

All anaesthetists should be able to: recognise and treat the patient at risk of cardiac arrest recognise and call for help if cardiac arrest occurs . Start cardiopulmonary resuscitation (CPR) based on current guidelines and attempt defibrillation if indicated.

Postoperative management:

Airway obstruction •

Hypoxia •

Haemorrhage: internal or external •

Hypotension and/or hypertension •

Postoperative pain • Shivering, hypothermia •

Vomiting, aspiration •

Falling on the floor •

Residual narcosis

The recovering patient is fit for the ward when: •

Awake, opens eyes • Extubated •

Blood pressure and pulse are satisfactory •

Can lift head on command •

Not hypoxic •

Breathing quietly and comfortably •

Appropriate analgesia has been prescribed and is safely established

Post operative pain relief (continued) •

Ideal way to give analgesia postoperatively is to: o Give a small intravenous bolus of about a quarter or a third of the maximum dose (e.g. 25 mg pethidine or 2.5 mg morphine for an average adult) o Wait for 5–10 minutes to observe the effect: the desired effect is analgesia, but retained consciousness o Estimate the correct total dose (e.g. 75 mg pethidine or 7.5 mg morphine) and give the balance intramuscularly. o

With this method, the patient receives analgesia quickly and the correct dose is given • If opiate analgesia is needed on the ward, it is most usual to give an intramuscular regimen: ¾ Morphine: – Age 1 year to adult: 0.1–0.2 mg/kg – Age 3 months to 1 year: 0.05–0.1 mg/kg ¾ Pethidine: give 7–10 times the above doses if using pethidine • Opiate analgesics should be given cautiously if the age is less than 1 year.

They are not recommended for babies aged less than 3 months unless very close monitoring in a neonatal intensive care unit is available. Anaesthesia & Pain Control in Children • Ketamine anaesthesia is widely used for children in rural centres (see pages 14–14 to 14–21), but is also good for pain control. • Children suffer from pain as much as adults, but may show it in different ways. •

Make surgical procedures as painless as possible: o Oral paracetamol can be given several hours prior to operation o Local anaesthetics (bupivacaine 0.25%, not to exceed 1 ml/kg) administered in the operating room can decrease incisional pain o Paracetamol (10–15 mg/kg every 4–6 hours) administered by mouth or rectally is a safe and effective method for controlling postoperative pain o For more severe pain, use intravenous narcotics (morphine sulfate 0.05–0.1 mg/kg IV) every 2–4 hours o Ibuprofen 10 mg/kg can be administered by mouth every 6–8 hours o Codeine suspension 0.5–1 mg/kg can be administered by mouth every 6 hours, asWHO/EHT/CPR: WHO Surgical Care at the District Hospital 2003.

Suggested reading:

1. Saravanan P, Soar J. A survey of resuscitation training needs of senior anaesthetists. Resuscitation 2005;64:93–96. 2

2. Soar J et al; Education, Implementation, and Teams Chapter Collaborators. Part 12: Education, implementation, and teams: 2010 International Consensus on Cardiopulmonary Resuscitation and Emergency Cardiovascular Care Science with Treatment Recommendations. Resuscitation 2010;81 (Suppl 1):e288–330. 3 Soar J et al. European Resuscitation Council Guidelines for Resuscitation 2010. Section 9. Principles of education in resuscitation. Resuscitation 2010;81:1434–1444.

3. Nolan JP et al; on behalf of the ERC Guidelines Writing Group. European Resuscitation Council Guidelines for Resuscitation 2010: Section 1.

4. February 2010 The Good Anaesthetist Standards of Practice for Career Grade Anaesthetists The Royal College of Anaesthetists The Association of Anaesthetists of Great Britain and Ireland ISBN: 978-1-900936-00-2 Published February 2010

5. WHO/EHT/CPR: WHO Surgical Careat the District Hospital 200

6. www.radiology.upmc.edu/MRsafety/
   A Web site developed by Dr.Emanuel Kanal, Chair of the American College of Radiology Blue Ribbon Panel on MR Safety. Includes other links.

7. www.fda.gov/cdrh/index.html
   FDA home page for medical devices. No specific listing exists for 'MR Compatible Devices"

8. http://www.simplyphysics.com/
   Educational products and photos of unusual projectiles.

9. www.acr.org/dyna/?doc=frames/main-sitemap.html
   MR safe practice guidelines by the American College of Radiology.

10. Jonathan R Treadwell, PhD and Scott Lucas, PhD, PE. Making Health Care Safer II: An Updated Critical Analysis of the Evidence for Patient Safety Practices. Chapter 13Preoperative Checklists and Anesthesia Checklists

11. Checklist for anaesthetic equipment 2012. Anaesthesia 2012; 66: pages 662–63.
    http://onlinelibrary.wiley.com/doi/10.1111/j.1365-2044.2012.07163.x/abstract

12. Immunization of Health-Care Workers: Recommendations of the Advisory Committee on Immunization Practices (ACIP) and the Hospital Infection Control Practices Advisory Committee (HICPAC)

www.ingramcontent.com/pod-product-compliance
Lightning Source LLC
Chambersburg PA
CBHW071019180526
45168CB00003B/1481